Bees & Other Stinging Insects

Bee Aware and *Bee* Safe

Another book from the
10 things to know™
series, companion to
Bees & Other
Stinging Insects
Bee Aware and *Bee* Safe

———————————————

Poison Ivy, Pets, & People
*Scratching the Poison Ivy, Oak,
and Sumac Itch*

———————————————

Bees & Other Stinging Insects
Bee Aware and *Bee* Safe

Heidi Ratner-Connolly
and
Randy Connolly

Book Design by Heidi Ratner-Connolly
ISBN 0-9722400-0-4
Published by 2LAKES PUBLISHING
Distributed by IPG/Chicago Review Press

Acknowledgements: We would like to thank our friend
and editor, Martha Tenney, for helping to enhance our
books and bring them to fruition.

CONTENTS

Introduction

The 1st Thing You Need to Know

Going *Bee*-neath the Surface

The 2nd Thing You Need to Know

Bee-twixt and *Bee*-tween

The 3rd Thing You Need to Know

Bee-yond the Itch

The 4th Thing You Need to Know

Bee-ing Prepared

The 5th Thing You Need to Know

Bee-ware the Sting

The 6th Thing You Need to Know

Bee-low the Skin

The 7th Thing You Need to Know

Bee Treated to *Bee* Sure

The 8th Thing You Need to Know

The *Bee*-nevolent Bee

The 9th Thing You Need to Know

Bee-yond the Traditional

The 10th Thing You Need to Know

Bee-ing Careful and Consciencious

INTRODUCTION

"Just *Bee*-tween Us..."

If you're anything like I am, you adore the warmer weather and what it brings...flowers, sunshine, ocean wading and BBQ's. But there is always that niggling fear that appears along with the first buds and the taste of watermelon..."Oh, no, it's THAT time of year again." That's right...the time for bees, wasps, hornets and mosquitos. The time when nature threatens to disturb the lovely peace of hiking, gardening or rocking on the porch swing.

The Story Behind the Story

When I was young, I sat on a rock. Unfortunately, there was a wasp on the rock, so I also sat on the wasp. (Believe me, I would not make this up.) The wasp was clearly put out and stung me with a vengeance you-know-where.

That is the first time I can remember seeing a part of my body (that shall remain nameless) swollen like a balloon. And that was the beginning of my lifelong fear of stinging insects.

As I grew up, I realized that stings and bites of all kinds were not simply an inconvenience, as they were for most people I knew. The swelling, itching, pain and nausea I experienced kept me from experiencing some of life's basic pleasures. Especially combined with my sensitivity to poison ivy and sumac, things like hiking became less than appealing. Overnight camp was a definite "challenge." As my mother used to say (and as your mother may have said to you), when you would ask why you were the one they chose to bite or sting, "That's because you're so sweet and tasty." Some consolation.

It seems that allergies tend to run in families and, in fact, my younger sister carries around an "*Epi-pen*" (a medical treatment discussed more fully in Chapter VII) after the time her lungs and legs 'blew up' from the sting of a bee. My older sister relocated to an entirely different climate to get away from her severe pollen allergies. My mother—well, the list is too long for this kind of book! And then there's my husband and me…stinging insects, dust, poison ivy, medicines…let's just say we're very sensitive people!

What I'm trying to say in this roundabout way is that if you happen to have any of these sensitivities yourself, or you know someone who does, you live just a little differently from "other" people—you're just a little more wary, just a little more circumspect about what you do, how you do it, and where you do it.

On the other hand, our fears are encouraged beyond all logic when we read about how "killer bees attack entire family..." or similar exaggerated stories. So, what we hope this book will do is give you back a little of your joie de vivre, your freedom, and your passions. Once you know the facts about these little flying torpedoes, and once you know the risks not to take, when the time comes that you are actually around them, your fears will—well, maybe not disappear completely, but certainly *bee* alleviated.

The 1st Thing to Know

Going *Bee*-neath the Surface

Hymenoptera

"Hymenoptera"—is that the name of a Greek god? A fancy dessert? No. It's just a scientific term (and one of the few used in this book!) for the estimated 300,000 species of stinging insects in the world. Not a *bee*guiling thought, eh? And only 120,000 of these insects have been identified and named so far!

Hymenoptera are simply insects that cause "allergy." (For those who like scientific terms, another word for allergy is "anaphylaxis.") There are many types of allergy-causing insects (many, many more than the average—yet sensitive—person would care to imagine), but we can save ourselves time by mentioning the ones with which we in the United States come in contact the most: all types of bees, yellow jackets and other types of wasps, hornets and fire ants (in certain parts of the country). And that should be enough to get our education going.

Human Statistics

"Lots of people die from stings, right?" Well, not really, comparatively…

It is estimated that between one and two million people in the United States are severely allergic to stinging insect venom. Each year 90 to 100 deaths from sting reactions are reported, but it's possible that many more deaths may actually be occurring, mistakenly diagnosed as heart attacks and sunstrokes or attributed to other causes. These stings include those by wasps, yellow jackets and bees.

Bee Alert!

Stinging insects play a vital part in our environment and economy. When we confuse them by wearing bright colors and sweet scents, cover picnic tables with our food supply, etc., they are attracted to us and our surroundings. When we threaten them, they aggressively protect themselves and their hives. They are very unlikely to sting until they perceive a threat, however. Our best protection is not to poison or bait, but to respect their habits and give them the wide berth that they deserve. Then stings become a much rarer occurrence.

Let's take a look at some common questions and answers before moving ahead.

Why do some of us seem to attract stinging insects more than others?...

And why do some of us get stung more than others? More men than women get stung, and while I doubt it's because men are tastier, it could be because males come into contact with stinging insects more often due to occupational and recreational exposure. With the current ever-changing career force, wouldn't it be interesting to note if this phenomenon has been changing over time?

How many types of stinging insects are there?

There are many, MANY types of stinging insects. Fire ants alone are reputed to sting nine million Americans each year! In 1989, 32 people in the southern part of the United States died from the stings of these minute creatures. Presently fire ants make their homes solely in the Southeastern United States.

How do they sting?

Envenomation is the word describing how venom of the insect is inserted into the flesh of a human or animal. Members of the Hymenoptera "clan" envenomate us enough to be a major cause of morbidity and mortality, accounting for more fatalities than any other venomous animal.

Here are some stinging statistics to mull over:

- Over two million Americans are allergic to stinging insects.

- More than 500,000 people enter hospital emergency rooms every year suffering from insect stings, and 50 to 100 people die as a result of an allergic reaction to these stings. We can look at this fact two ways: first, 40 to 50 out of 500,000 is not a "relatively" high number. But, second, 100 people a year dying from insect stings is 100 people too many. Knowing the facts about treating stings quickly can save a life!

- Allergic reactions to insect stings usually occur very quickly after the sting itself—from within a few minutes up to 24 hours.

- People who have experienced a systemic allergic reaction to an insect sting have a 60% chance of a similar (or worse) reaction if stung again.

- Stinging insects are most active during the summer and early fall. Why? Because that's when their nest populations are at their highest levels, and can exceed 60,000 insects.

Bee-lieve It or Not!

More people die each year from the effects of insect venom than from either spider or snake bites.

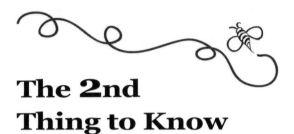

The 2nd
Thing to Know

Bee-twixt & *Bee*-tween
(*Hymenoptera*, the Species)

Hymenoptera—The Family

Bees and wasps are what I call first cousins in the *Hymenoptera* family. Bees seem to get the most press when it comes to stings. But wasps, the group that includes the hornet, can also pack a wallop. All these insects have a lot in common, notably their sting, but they also vary in distinct ways.

WASPS: Wasps tend to have much more aggressive natures than the usual honeybee, but the biggest difference between bees and wasps/hornets is that wasps can sting you multiple times in rapid succession! Why? They have a smooth kind of covering on their stingers which can be inserted and removed altogether too easily—again and again. *(See Photo Gallery Pages)*

The Stinging Difference...

Did you hear about the recent fad for "pheromones"? Those scents one can buy to drive the object of your desire crazy with passion? Well, pheromones are exactly what wasps uniquely use to attract others of their species to help them attack their victims. The pheromone is in the venom they inject and acts as a kind of loudspeaker to their friends and families, telling them to come over and partake in the action. We tend to think of bees acting in this manner—swarming, etc., but *bee* forewarned, because though we often see a single solitary wasp or hornet buzzing around, its solo status is deceiving. One angry wasp can send the call out to many more.

Types of Bees and Wasps

- Paper wasps are the least aggressive of all the wasps. They are more red and brown than yellow and black, and are usually found in more rural areas.

- Yellow jackets are known for their bright colors. Though pleasing in appearance, they are aggressive and found nearly everywhere, especially in northern temperate areas.

> • Hornets are brown and/or black and look as if they've been stuck together in pieces. They have yellow markings on their face and thorax. They too can be very aggressive.

There are two main kinds of bees:

The European Honey Bee, which includes the Africanized version in the United States, and the Bumblebee. There are also bee variations, such as the carpenter bee and the mud bee.

Africanized bees are currently confined to the more southern states in the United States. Attacks are infrequent, and these bees are actively sought out for destruction in this country.

What happens to the insect after the sting?

Wasps do not die after stinging their victims as bees do. They go on to sting another day—and another victim—or even the same victim yet again. This goes back to the fact that it is the bee that has the barbed stinger. Not only can it only sting once, but it cannot pull out the stinger after stinging.

For bees, on the other hand, death is definitely not *bee*-coming. Once it has stung its victim, the bee has to literally rip itself from its stinger, still connected to its venom *sac*. The venom continues to pump into the victim's system for up to a minute. The bee, having left part of itself *bee*-hind in its victim, flies off and dies a *bee*-lated death.

How does the sting really sting?

All these insects inject the venom just the way a doctor injects fluid into a patient using a syringe. The venom has to this point been stored in the insect's abdomen.

Bee-lieve It or Not!

Let's not forget fire ants. These creatures attack humans with relish, but will do just about anything to resist attack themselves, especially by a tiny fly called the phorid that measures only about one-sixteenth of an inch. This fly—females only—actually pierces the fire ant's head and then releases an enzyme that later decapitates it!

Once the "stinger" is inserted into the skin, the venom begins to squirt into the tube-like stinger. Actually, the stinger is an evolved part of the female insect's egg-laying organ. And this is the reason that only females of the species (both bees and wasps) can sting.

But now, back to our wasp who is continuing to sting and re-sting her victim. It is not a pretty picture, really, to describe how the wasp "stings." In reality, "sting" is a misnomer, because the wasp thrusts its shaft-like stinger into the victim and the blade moves rapidly backwards and forwards in a sawing-type action. I repeat, this description is not for the fainthearted.

The "blades" have what are like little jagged teeth along their edges. As the stinger goes deeper into the victim's body, the edges grip the flesh until the other blades can move forward so the shaft goes deeper and deeper into the wound. The movement of the blades causes a kind of pumping action to occur at the end of the shaft which then causes the poison sac to pump venom down through a central canal.

But what happens to ME?

RIGHT...That's what happens to the stingers, but what happens to the "stingees?" Here's what actually happens when you get stung.

Single stings: Stingers are effective weapons be-cause they deliver a venom that causes pain when injected into the skin, stimulating the nerve endings of the pain receptors. The major chemical responsible for the pain of a honeybee sting is called Melittin. As some of us unfortunately know all too well, the result is pain, starting as a sharp pain and then becoming a dull ache. In my own experiences, the sting location stays sore and tender for days afterwards—if not longer.

How does the body respond?

When we're stung, our bodies send fluid from our blood directly to the site of the sting to try to flush out the venom from the area. That's why there is redness and swelling at the site of the sting. Hopefully, the swelling stays localized and does not lead to larger swelling of other areas of the body. The only good thing I can think of about being stung more than once in one's life is that if you have been stung more than once, your immune system is likely to recognize the venom and it will potentially be discarded more quickly.

So, back to the sting. The local area around the sting starts to itch. And of course it is generally agreed that the one thing we should NOT do it scratch it. It might feel like the thing to do, but scratching can sometimes bring bacteria into the wound and infection can set in.

What to do if or when you do get stung

Remove the stinger FAST. As you read earlier, a bee's stinger is basically ripped from the bee's body and will remain in *our* bodies until removed. Removing the stinger quickly is a good idea, because venom will continue to enter the skin for up to a minute. (We'll cover how to remove the stinger in a minute, but the most important thing to know is that you should remove it ASAP.) It's been shown that removing a stinger within 15 seconds of the sting can reduce its intensity considerably.

Removing the stinger

Again, it is very important to remove the stinger as early as possible. It is best to remove it with a pair of tweezers, but if tweezers aren't at hand it can be done by scraping it with a fingernail or the tip of a knife. Never squeeze the venom sac of the stinger, because more venom will enter the wound.

More sting removal tips

Okay, so now we've discussed removing the stinger ASAP. But there's a process for doing this that will make things look much brighter in the morning.

(1) **Locate the stinger.** You will probably see an area of redness and swelling, and the stinger will be in

the center, looking like a little black dot. If you look with a magnifying glass you may even be able to see the sac of venom attached!

(2) Flick out the stinger. Don't squeeze the stinger because it will continue to inject more venom. Using your fingers to pull it out doesn't work well for this reason. So, carefully try to flick or scratch it out with your fingerNAIL or a pointed object. You could even use the edge of a credit card to flick it out, and where we may not all carry around a pair of tweezers, we are rarely out of screaming distance of a credit card.

(3) Apply compress. Once the stinger is removed, especially if the stings are to the areas of the head or neck, which are much more dangerous, apply ice or cold compresses immediately. Meat tenderizer is great for neutralizing the venom. None in your back pocket, eh? Well, baking soda works really well too. None of that either? Turn to our Chapter on Remedies for tips on what else would be good to carry around in your backpack or glovebox.

Hymenoptera *Bee*-havior

Under the heading of behavior is the aspect of socialization. Bees and wasps are called "social" because they tend to swarm, attacking in groups rather than alone when disturbed.

The real problem is that if two or more attack (especially if they are wasps or hornets and can sting multiple times), mammals can be severely affected even if they are "non-allergic."

First, let's take a look at what *swarming* is really all about.

I was interested to learn that swarming takes place when the queen honeybee of the colony leaves the hive, followed by all the mature bees. They've left the younger bees behind who stay to do their job in raising a new queen. But I was surprised to learn that before the bees leave their nest, they get virtually "stoned" on honey, so really the idea is that they are a severe threat to us at that stage is somewhat of an exaggeration.

The bees then cluster around their queen at a suitable spot, such as on or in a log or on a branch. Scouts go off to find a good spot for the new nest and return to let everyone know the good news. Pretty soon they have all moved on to the new digs—unless, of course, they decided that your house is the perfect spot!

So, in essence, though swarming can be dangerous for us, the assumption that swarms are always "angry" is usually not a correct one.

The Not-So-Good-News About *Bee*-haviors

Let's compare the various species of Hymenoptera. Generally speaking, bees do not tend to be as aggressive as wasps/hornets. (It is true, however, that because there are more Africanized honeybees in the United States, this more aggressive type has inflicted more stings.)

Africanized bees actually have less venom than other bees, so technically you might be tempted to call them less dangerous. However, although they are less malevolent when by their "onesies," they are also extremely sensitive and testy as a group, seeming to have a one-for-all and all-for-one mentality. Needless to say, this works wonders as a defensive policy.

Africanized bees exhibit *socialized* traits, and may swarm and defend their nests when approached from up to 150 yards away. They have been known to chase after intruders for miles—even in their cars! I do not advocate for the extermination of any creature, but these bees are not only dangerous to human beings, but also tend to drive away our good-natured (or should we say "less aggressively-natured") honeybees.

Wasps tend to be more aggressive than bees in general and may sting more often; however, more people are allergic to bee venom than to wasp/hornet venom.

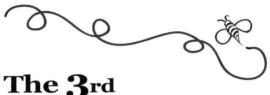

The 3rd Thing to Know

Bee-yond the Itch

Allergic Reactions

Let's begin by addressing a few basic facts that can be confusing.

What does it mean to be "allergic?"

Part of the confusion here seems to stem from the fact that many of us talk about "being allergic" when what we're describing is any type of reaction we have from eating something, getting stung by something etc. Another word for allergy is "anaphylaxis" (as in *anaphylactic shock*). For example, my son regularly told his friends' parents he was allergic to tomatoes so he wouldn't have to eat them. How convenient.

However, having a "reaction" to something simply means the food, the sting, the dust mite or whatever it is causes a local reaction, such as a welt on the skin and a period of itching or sneezing.

This is different from "being allergic" or having an "allergic reaction," meaning having a systemic reaction, one that travels through the body, for example to the heart, and one that can be fatal. Going back to my sister's allergy to bees for a minute, her reaction causes the area of the sting to swell instantly and then start to travel throughout the body. Without quick medical intervention, her lungs are in danger of closing off.

The following descriptions should help you get an idea about which reaction might be the one to worry about.

- **A "normal" reaction** to an insect sting only lasts a few hours. That's not to say that it doesn't hurt. The sting site will be painful; it will probably be red and swollen and may even drive you to the emergency room. These symptoms, however, under "normal" conditions, will quickly subside.

- **A local reaction** that is somewhat more severe in nature will last for several days. The pain and swelling will stay around longer and cause you more angst!

- **A "severe" allergic reaction** is the one we all hear about, the one where limbs swell and hives break out, the person may feel dizzy, nauseated and/or weak. Some even have stomach cramps and diarrhea. Others have been known to itch around the eyes, have a "warm" feeling, vomit, cough, or have darkened skin.

The whole body will be affected during a severe reaction. This is the one to watch for when you or someone else has been stung. The symptoms can begin very rapidly, usually within five minutes, and most deaths from stings occur within thirty. Some deaths have actually been reported to have taken place in five to fifteen minutes.

Do our allergic reactions get worse over time?

Most health care providers agree that once a person has had a severe reaction, it usually increases in severity with each new sting. More severe reactions tend to occur in people whose onset of symptoms was especially fast.

The allergic element of the venom

The venom differs between species, but in humans it is generally found that the allergic element of the venom falls into two categories: bees or wasp/hornet venom. It is quite common for individuals to be allergic to one venom and not the other.

"You'll grow out of it."

Another misconception about stinging insects is that children are more susceptible to experiencing stronger reactions than their adult counterparts. People generally believe this about many types of allergies, signified by the old adage, "You'll grow out of it." In fact, the older you are, the worse it gets! (And, no, I'm not talking about wrinkles or gravity, either!)

Stings are reported to occur more often in adults than in children, and the reactions are generally more severe. One common theory is that this is because adults have had more time/opportunity to develop a higher sensitivity to the allergens in the insect's venom.

It is also true, however, that when a child *does* develop an allergic reaction, that reaction will tend to be much worse than an adult's initial onset reaction. Why? The accepted theory behind that fact is that there is a higher ratio of venom to body mass in a child than in an adult.

Stings and Children

Are you concerned that one or more of your children could be allergic to stinging insects? If you are, and you'll never know for sure unless it happens, unfortunately, take the available precautions (such as seeing an allergist), and make preparations in advance in the event of a sting occurring. And always talk to your health care provider about these kinds of medical issues well in advance.

If you are allergic...

People who are known to be allergic to wasps and bees should try wherever and whenever possible to avoid being stung and stay away from areas frequented by bees and wasps (of course, you say!).

But, if or when a wasp or bee approaches, it is still the best policy to remain calm and still, and not try to swat the insect as this may frighten it. If it lands on you, gently blow it off your skin.

Remember, attraction often relates to smell, and things that smell good to us also smell good to the bees (and other buzzing things). So let's start with what I call the "Avoidance Theory," which simply says, "Staying away from stinging insects is the best sure way to avoid getting stung!" Not rocket science, admittedly, but it's definitely the way to get started. The gamut of allergic reactions runs something like this:

- hives or itching
- swelling at other than the sting site
- difficulty breathing
- dizziness
- nausea
- cramps
- diarrhea
- unconsciousness
- cardiac arrest

Just to Reiterate...

An allergic reaction to an insect sting can occur immediately, within minutes, or even up to 24 hours. Here is a list of the common potential allergic reactions:

Africanized Bees and Allergic Reactions

As mentioned in the last chapter, Africanized bees have almost 30% less venom than regular European honeybees. So, though their venom itself is less, well, venomous, they are definitely NOT less dangerous because of their aggressive nature when in groups.

The **4**th Thing to Know

Bee-ing Prepared

Prevention

Let's set the scene...

Joan and John go for a picnic. From the minute they approach the lovely field full of wildflowers (a truly romantic spot), Joan is *bee*-sieged by buzzing insects around her body and head. John is meandering along the same path without incident. Joan begins to panic because the insects do not seem to leave her alone. John wants to lie down and have a snooze before lunch.

So, why do some people attract stinging insects more than others? Do we wear signs that say, "I'm here, look at me, I love to be annoyed, bothered and stung?" (For that matter, do bees read?)

As we mentioned earlier, men do get stung more than women, possibly because they are outdoors more while working. And some people are just more allergic than others. However, we also know that there are a number of things that stimulate hymenoptera to come a-callin'.

First, let's cover the general avoidance techniques we might all want to practice...**BECAUSE PREVENTION IS BY FAR THE BEST POLICY.**

Avoidance

> • **Clothes.** Always avoid bright colors. Stinging insects are attracted to bright colors specifically. However, though you might consider white a "bright" color, it is actually the best color to wear. Avoid shiny buckles and jewelry. Wear a hat and closed shoes (not sandals). It may surprise you to hear that loose-fitting clothing is not a good idea either, because it may attract and then trap the insects. Hymenoptera seem to have

good taste also; flowery prints and black are extremely motivating.

- Beekeepers wear their own version of bee-safe clothes, including light colors of cotton—never wool. Beginning beekeepers go so far as to add bee gloves, a head veil, long sleeves and coveralls with the pant legs tucked into boots or tied at the ankles to prevent multiple stings.

- **Scents.** Avoid wearing perfumes, aftershaves, colognes and don't use scented soaps. This is a tough one, because most everything we put on our bodies these days is scented. And most of them are scented with flower scents—the worst kind if you're hoping to avoid insects. You really have to make an effort and search our shampoos, conditioners and soaps that specifically say "unscented."

- **Don't go barefoot.**

- **Don't swat** or otherwise provoke bees or yellow jackets with your bare hands.

- **Check** in and around the moist or damp beach towel you left on the lounge chair before you pick it up...insects just love to find a little place in there to soak up the moisture.

- **Always keep foods covered.** Drinking from open containers is especially hazardous because insects can be hidden inside. Outdoor cooking, feeding pets, etc., are like ringing the dinner bell for an entire family—and their relatives!

- **Soda cans** act as little beacons to a stinging insects...they zoom right in to the smell of the sugar. Yellow jackets are drawn to soft drinks BIG-TIME. Fruit juices are just as appealing.

- **Suntan lotion** is another bad idea for the sting-prone individual. The smell of coconut is pretty common in today's lotions, but besides making one dream of pina coladas, it drives the hymenoptera crazy with desire!

- **Shake out any clothing** you've left lying on the ground. Insects are easily hidden and easily aggravated if you happen to put them on along with your shirt or shoes.

For those of us who verge on paranoia, here's a more extensive list of DON'Ts!

- Don't stick your finger into **flowers**. (This may be better reserved for younger children, but one never knows.) Insects are hidden inside collecting pollen.

- **Clover** covered lawns look oh-so-soft and barefoot-able, but don't be tempted. Insects especially love that clover...and dandelions, too.

- It's not a good idea to **mow grass**, trim hedges or prune trees in mid-summer. That's the unfortunate fact.

- Bees and wasps are drawn to **picnic areas**, clover fields, etc., by their natures. They do not need to be helped along by uncovered foods, soft drinks or garbage containers. Rotting fruit on the ground is another feast to a stinging insect.

- Never disturb a beehive you happen upon. You might think it's common sense, but hives can look rather deserted, that is until you start to poke and prod them.

- Stinging insects are most dangerous when you—and they—are close to their nests. Anyone passing by can be considered a threat to the safety of their home. What would you do if

> someone threatened your family and home? Right, chase them away...in this case, with a sting.

So, when you meet a bee?...FLEE! If you do happen to come across a swarm of bees, run for shelter. Bees are actually slow flyers and normally you will be able to outrun them.

Bees also fly in straight lines. It's amazing but true. What's the problem with that? They are busy flying between their pollen source (flowers) and their hives and tend to collide with anything in their path. In other words, you and me, the unsuspecting obstacles.

Words of Wisdom

If a wasp or bee approaches, STAY STILL!!! I know it's probably the hardest thing to do—it is for me, anyway, but do not try to swat away the insect. This will only frighten it or aggravate it. If it does happen to land on you, gently try to blow it off your skin.

You can also slowly raise your arms to protect your face, and then move **S-L-O-W-L-Y** away to escape indoors. Moving RAPIDLY provokes attack.

NEVER strike or swing at a wasp or bee, pushing it against your body. If you inadvertently trap it against you, it may sting you out of fear.

And don't forget the really bad part—if you crush a wasp, or it stings you, the pheromones released could incite many, many more to come back and attack with frenzy. You definitely don't want hundreds of "guard wasps" zooming in for the kill.

It's also a real test of your ability to stay calm if you find a bee or a wasp has thumbed a ride in your car. But that's exactly what you should do. STAY CALM. Of course, the insect doesn't really want to be there much

BEE-lieve It or Not!

Did you know that bees tend to be more angry on cloudy, dark, rainy days in early spring of the year?

either and would prefer another way to travel. They usually fly against the windows in the car trying to get out. They rarely sting the occupants unless agitated (the insects, not the people).

The best thing to do is to slowly and safely pull off the road, open the window and allow the bee or wasp to escape.

Because it is so hard to stay focused on your driving with a stinging insect about, serious accidents often occur when drivers reflexively swing their arms at the insect.

Advice for the Allergic or Hypersensitive

Don't take risks. If you know you are allergic or even hypersensitive, you should never be alone when hiking, boating, swimming, golfing, fishing or doing anything else outdoors. This is simply because if you are stung, you will likely need someone else's immediate help to start FAST emergency treatment.

It's a good idea to carry some form of ID card, bracelet or necklace (such as "Medic Alert") which will identify you as allergic to stings in an emergency situation. You may have gone into sudden anaphylactic shock or have fainted, particularly if you've been stung more than once. (See *Reference* pages for information on procuring a device from the Medic Alert Foundation.)

The 5th Thing to Know

Bee-ware the Sting

Avoidance Tips—The Short List

Knowing how to avoid stings from bees, wasps, hornets and yellow jackets leads to a more enjoyable day for everyone. This list of suggestions is a culmination of many, many lists we read in our research.

> 1. Avoid walking barefoot in the grass. Honeybees and bumblebees forage on white clover, a weed that grows in lawns throughout the United States.
>
> 2. Insect repellents DO NOT work against stinging insects.

3. Never swat or flail at a flying insect. If need be, gently brush it aside or patiently wait for it to leave.

4. DO NOT drink from open beverage cans. Stinging insects will crawl inside a can attracted by the sweet beverage.

5. When eating outdoors, try to keep food covered at all times. Stinging insects are fond of the same foods you are.

6. Garbage cans stored outside should be covered with tight-fitting lids.

7. Avoid wearing sweet-smelling per-fumes, hair sprays, colognes, and deodorants.

8. Avoid wearing bright-colored cloth-ing with flowery patterns. Bees may mistake you for a flower.

Stinging Insects
Are Smart, So...

Don't scream. This only irritates the insects more and will increase the attack's ferociousness.

Don't run towards other people. They will also get attacked.

Don't hide under water. Sometimes these insects wait until you surface for air and then— WATCH OUT!

The **6**th
Thing to Know

Bee-low the Skin

Getting Stung

Let's take time to delve a little more deeply into what actually happens when you get stung by any kind of hymenoptera, so any misconceptions you may have will clear up.

What does the actual stinging process entail?

Stingers are effective weapons because the venom they deliver causes pain when it's injected into the skin. The major chemical responsible for the pain of a honey bee sting is called Melittin which stimulates the nerve endings of pain receptors in the skin. The result is a very painful sensation, which begins as a sharp pain that lasts a few minutes and then becomes a dull ache. Even up to a few days later, the tissue may still be sensitive to the touch (and I can personally vouch for that!).

What is the body's actual response?

The body responds to stings by liberating fluid from the blood to flush venom components from the area. This causes redness and swelling at the sting site. If this is not the first time that the person has been stung by that species of insect, it is likely that the immune system will recognize the venom and enhance the disposal procedure. This can lead to a very large area of swelling around the sting site or in a whole portion of the body. The area is quite likely to itch.

Oral and topical antihistamines should help prevent or reduce the itching and swelling. Try not to rub or scratch the sting site because microbes from the surface of the skin could be introduced into the wound and result in an infection.

> • When the sting is caused by a honey-bee, the stinger usually remains in the skin when the insect leaves because the stinger is barbed. Removing the stinger as quickly as possible is the key here, because

venom continues to enter the skin from the stinger for 45 to 60 seconds following a sting. Much has been written about the proper way to remove a bee stinger, but new information indicates that it doesn't matter how you get it out as long as it is removed as soon as possible, and without squeezing it. If removed within 15 seconds of the sting, the severity of the sting is reduced.

- After the sting is removed, wash the wound and treat it. It may not be a good idea to exercise or have a hot bath after a sting as this could increase the venom distribution.

Controlling the Pain of a Sting

You can use over-the-counter products or a simple cold compress or ice pack to control the pain of a sting. (For more information see Chapters VII and XIX.)

When to seek medical attention

If the sting is followed by severe symptoms, or if it occurs on the neck or mouth, seek medical attention immediately because swelling in these areas of the body can cause suffocation.

Single vs. multiple stings or "mass envenomation"

Occasionally, a person is stung many times before being able to flee from a nesting site or the site of attack. Depending on the number of stings, the person may just hurt a lot, feel a little sick, or feel very sick. Humans can be killed if stung enough times in a single incident.

In this particular situation, children are clearly at a greater risk than adults. In fact, if you are an otherwise healthy adult, you would have to be stung about 1,000 times for death to be a risk (*without* a systemic reaction). Most deaths caused by multiple stings have occurred in men in their 70's or 80's with histories of heart or other dysfunction.

More Serious Conditions

It is not our goal to frighten any of our readers, but we believe it's important to provide the whole picture (albeit in short form). There is another potentially life-threatening condition that results from multiple stings and which can occur days after the incident. This condition is called *renal insufficiency*. Suffice it to say that proteins in the venom damage the cells and keep debris that would naturally be eliminated through the kidneys from being eliminated. If the kidneys become clogged, the person is in danger of kidney failure and death.

So, again, don't take one sting or multiple stings lightly. Go to your health care provider for either bee or wasp stings and discuss/monitor potential secondary effects that could happen over time.

DON'T
—WE REPEAT—
DON'T:

Scream. This only irritates the insects more and will increase the attack's ferociousness.

Run towards other people. They will also get attacked.

Hide under water. Sometimes these insects wait until you surface for air and then—WATCH OUT!

The 7th Thing to Know

Bee Treated to *Bee* Sure

Medical & Conventional Treatments

It's probably the most natural thing in the world to go see an allergist once you've already had an allergic reaction to an insect sting. Unfortunately, if you haven't ever had a reaction, you don't know what your chances are of being the person who just gets red and swollen or the person who will have a more systemic reaction.

Our opinion is that if you have a family member who is allergic or you believe you may be allergic for any other reason (perhaps you have many other allergies), you might want to see an allergist to learn for certain.

In fact, if you have had a reaction before, you have a 60% chance of having a similar or worse reaction if stung again.

Insect Kits

Very often, if it turns out you are allergic, the allergist will recommend you carry an insect sting treatment kit wherever you go. Insect "treatment kits" utilize *epinephrine injectors*. People who are highly allergic to stinging insects often carry this kind of medication with them at all times, available just in case the unexpected happens.

- *Anakits* or *Epi-pens* are two types that are available on-line or at pharmacies. Administering the medication correctly is critical, so make sure you know how to use the kit before you actually need it. It's always best to follow the manufacturer's directions to the letter. Naturally, even if you use the kit, seek out medical attention as quickly as possible in case further treatment is necessary.

- Kits are expensive, as well as potentially dangerous, and their potential use should always be discussed in advance with your health care provider.

- It's best to try to keep two emergency kits ready and with you at all times. Sometimes one in your purse, briefcase or knapsack, and one in your car works well too. However, because kits should be stored in a cool, dry place, the car may not always be the best place. Do the best you can with the circumstances you have.

- These kits usually contain one sterile syringe of epinephrine (adrenaline) ready for injection, four chewable, yellow tablets of Chlortrimetron (antihistamine), two sterile alcohol swabs for cleaning the injection site, and one tourniquet.

Precise use of the kit will not be discussed here, as that information is best discussed with your health care provider. Some providers recommend adrenaline inhalers to relieve chest tightness and throat swelling, and are available by injection or orally.

> With honeybees, the toxic dose of the venom is estimated to be 8.6 stings per pound of body weight.

Venom Immunotherapy

There are varying statistics about the effectiveness of venom immunotherapy in preventing future allergic reactions to insect stings. However, the authors have read that it can be up to 97% effective for some people. (See the next chapter for more information on this fascinating subject.)

The 8th Thing to Know

The *Bee*-nevolent Bee

Bees and Their Products

Though I make a concerted effort to dodge stinging insects, I also appreciate that honeybees hold a special place in our universe. In fact, the medicinal use of honey products has been practiced since ancient times. Chinese physicians 4000 years ago used *apitherapy*, the practice of using bee pollen and other bee products for therapeutic uses, commonly.

As early as 130 A.D., the Roman physician Galen prescribed *Bee Venom Therapy* (BVT) and the famous Charlemagne was known to use bee stings to mitigate symptoms of arthritis. In Athens, in 530 B.C., laws were written to protect apiaries based on the belief that they were so vital to Greek life.

In other words, using bees and their products for medicinal purposes has been going on for a very long time; we call it an "alternative therapy," but really it's the oldest therapy in the book!

Bee farms are known as *apiaries* and *apitherapy* is the practise of using bee pollen, propolis (sticky resin the bees collect from buds to protect their hives), royal jelly, beeswax, honey or bee venom for therapeutic use.

Honey bee venom is currently most frequently used to treat conditions such as:

- **Arthritis and other inflammatory and degenerative diseases** (including osteo- and rheumatoid arthritis). BVT helps with pain and swelling in these conditions.

- **Acute and chronic injuries,** such as bursitis and tendinitis. Again, the effect may be due to a localized anti-inflammatory reaction. Chronic back and neck pain have also been known to respond to this therapy.

- **Scar tissue**. Scar tissue can actually be broken down, softened, flattened out, and even begin to fade in color by the substances in the bee venom.

- **Multiple sclerosis**. Though undertaking this kind of bee therapy can be prolonged and difficult, many MS patients still seek it out because some of its benefits are reported to include better stability, less fatigue and fewer spasms. Patients sometimes insist that the therapy must be done for 6 months, 2 to 3 times per week, to give it a full test.

How does it work?

Without getting technical (and we are not medical professionals), bee venom contains more than 18 active substances. The highest concentration is of Melittin, a potent anti-inflammatory agent (100 times more than hydrocortisol). There are also other anti-inflammatory agents, plus one that blocks certain channels and enhances nerve transmission.

How is it done?

For over 60 years and until his recent death, one bee-keeper in Middlebury, Vermont, had used BVT for just about any situation where nothing else had worked. (Please note that the authors neither advocate nor oppose its use.) Many satisfied "patients" felt strongly that the therapy helped their conditions under his care, and others continue to follow suit.

BVT is undertaken by a beekeeper, by the patient him or herself, or even by the patient's partner who learns the technique. A bee is taken from the jar or hive, held over an area of the body with tweezers, and basically one just waits until the bee does its thing! It does sound pretty tough to just sit and wait for it to happen, doesn't it? And, depending on the nature of the problem and its length, one may need several stings in a sitting, two or three times per week, for several months.

What's in the bee venom?

Many flying insects have a venomous sting, but because the honeybee has been domesticated and is easy to raise, it is the one used most for treatment. Two of the components included in honeybee venom are:

> • **Mellitin**, which provides the "ouch" and the itch, along with the inflammation through the release of hista-

mine. On the positive side, it also stimulates the pituitary to release ACTH, which stimulates the adrenal glands to produce cortisol, and voila, the cortisol stimulates your body's own healing response.

Interestingly, Mellitin is also 100 times more potent as an anti-inflammatory agent than hydrocortisol—at least in arthritic rats (as reported in *Nature Magazine* in 1974).

- **Mast Cell Degranulating Peptide.** This substance also releases histamine which "helps" along the swelling, the itching, the redness and the warmth—basically, all the things that make you feel lousy.

  What's interesting about this substance is that it can induce seizures more powerfully than any other known substance. Is there a "good news" part? Well, it does seem to increase short-term memory in rats...we'll have to see about that one.

Can bee venom be taken orally?

We could not find much information on this topic, but in what we read there was nothing indicating that bee venom is available in capsules, tablets or other form.

There are, however, literally dozens of products in the homeopathic marketplace, especially in Europe. (See Chapter XIX for more information on homeopathic remedies.)

Are there injections of bee venom?

There are physicians around who use bee venom therapy in their practices. They obtain the venom in sterilized vials and inject it under the patient's skin, sometimes mixing it with an anesthetic. Some say that collecting the venom in vials makes it less potent, but it may be a viable option if you don't have access to beekeepers where you are!

There are a few ways to actually locate a bee-keeper—one who is willing to sting you on purpose.

> • Call local beekeepers and beekeeper organizations.
>
> • Contact the American Apitherapy Society, headquartered in Vermont.

PHOTO GALLERY

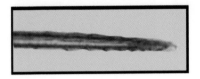

The bee's stinger is barbed. It hooks into its victim's flesh and rips away from the bee, who flies off and dies(above).

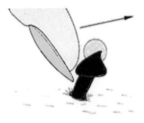

A sting can cause several levels of allergic reaction —from local (below) to systemic.

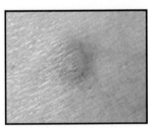

Flick the bee or wasp sting out with a fingernail or tweezers so it doesn't slide in further (above).

(Pictures and photographs courtesy of David Glaser)

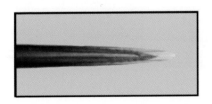

The wasp's stinger is smooth and can slide in and out easily, enabling the wasp to sting its victim more than once in rapid succession (left).

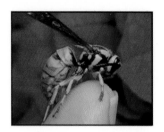 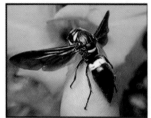

Giant hornet (left); Hornet (right)

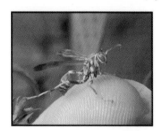 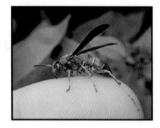

Paperwasps (above); Yellowjacket (below)

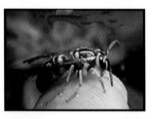

(Photos compliments of David Glaser)

Yellowjacket (left; Bald-faced Hornet (below)

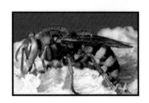 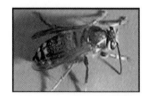

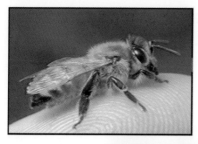

(Photos compliments of David Glaser)

Honeybees at work (top, right)

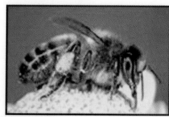

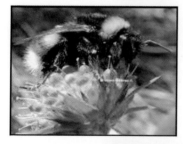

Bumblebee gathering pollen (left)

Carpenter bee sits calmly on photographer's finger (right)

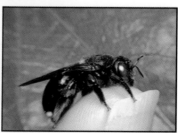

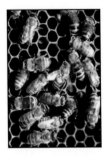

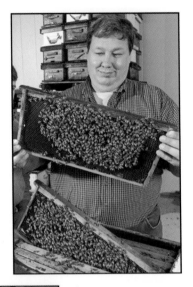

These bees have little brown bumps on their backs that are actually Varroa Jacobsoni *mites (above) (photo by Lila De Guzman).*

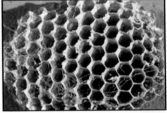

Checking the health of the bee colony at a bee farm (above) (photo by Stephen Ausmus).

Wasps nest (above). Giant Hornets nest (right) (Photos compliment of Tim Prouty).

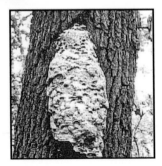

MS has always been described by Western medicine as *incurable*. In 1993, the drug *beta interferon* was put on the market with hopes of putting the disease into remission for certain patients. However, even with this kind of drug treatment, and aside from its expense, many people remain symptomatic.

BVT, though it has not been scientifically "proven" is relatively inexpensive and has (relatively) fewer and more minor side-effects. Because BVT is showing so much promise, the National MS Society is currently funding studies. The MS Society does NOT recommend this therapy yet, however, given the lack of evidence of its efficacy.

With all that said, responses to BVT seem as individual as the patients themselves. Some show improvement quickly, but others may take a longer period of time. Some may not improve at all. Unfortunately, the reasons for these variations are not yet understood.

What about bee venom and acupuncture?

Due to the long time usage of bee venom by Chinese acupuncturists (for at least three centuries), combined with the use of traditional acupuncture methods, BVT techniques have become more widespread and safer.

The Chinese have treated conditions such as epilepsy and impotency, along with the list of more commonly treated conditions mentioned earlier.

- Charles Mraz (deceased, 1999), formerly of Middlebury, Vermont, was a well-known source of wisdom and information on the topic of apitherapy. There is an on-going yearly conference in his name, and he wrote books on the subject for anyone interested in pursuing this topic. You may be reassured, as we were when we learned it, that bees are not killed or hurt in the collection of bee venom as they were in the past. Newer methods are both safe and economical.

What's the story with bee venom and multiple sclerosis?

MS patients' common symptoms are extreme fatigue, lack of balance, coordination and muscle control, as well as other neurologically based conditions, such as numbness. Progressive immobility is the norm.

Treating MS with live bee stings has a short history of only about a decade or so, and that is mostly anecdotal in nature. Given that fact, along with the lack of scientifically controlled studies, it is difficult to determine its true effectiveness.

An acupuncture needle can be dipped into the bee venom solution and then placed into the acupuncture points, or the solution can be placed directly on the body and then the needle inserted through the solution.

Are there uses for the other honeybee products?

There is anecdotal evidence that raw honey treats:

> - athlete's foot
> - conjunctivitis
> - topical fungal
> - infections
> - burns

Raw honey is also sometimes used:

> - for dressing cuts (based on its regenerative powers)
>
> - as a topical antibiotic
>
> - as a cold remedy (combined with apple cider vinegar and hot water).

An Un*bee*-lievable Story!

Two wasps (to be specific, their remains only) were found in the stomach of a dog. The tissue samples revealed that when the dog swallowed these wasps, they did not give up easily, evidenced by the stings down the very back of his tongue, throat and even down his esophagus. It seems that the poor dog suffered heart failure brought on by the anaphylactic shock following the multiple stings. At the time of death, his body temperature was 109F (shock can cause temperature spikes), which certainly could have led to the stroke.

A sad story to *bee*-hold, indeed.

The **9**th
Thing to Know

Bee-yond the Traditional

Homeopathic Remedies

It has often struck me that it's when we have no other options that we find a new way of doing things. Think about Tom Hanks in the movie *Castaway*. He certainly made due with the very little he could find on his deserted island to survive. When there's no drugstore around or no doctor's office or emergency room at hand immediately, what can you do?

Personally speaking, Randy and I are homeopathic enthusiasts and use many common remedies for many purposes. For some of our readers, it can simply be good to know the kinds of things that have helped other people at other times...just in case.

These herbal remedies have been researched from sites on the internet, including *www.Livingherbal.com*. They have not all been tried or tested by the authors and are not in any way suggested for use without careful consideration and/or the oversight of a health care professional.

The following products of nature have been used for centuries for bites and stings of all kinds.

- **Fendler Bladderpod.** Navajos used this treatment for spider bites when it was in the form of a tea.

- **Purple Coneflower.** The Plains Indians applied this remedy to treat all kinds of bites and stings and for all kinds of crawling, flying or leaping bugs.

- **Stiff Goldenrod.** For treating bee stings, the Meskwaki Indians of Minnesota ground up the goldenrod into a lotion. Since saliva is considered helpful also, chewing to grind leaves, etc., was a recommended course of action.

- **Trumpet Honeysuckle**. Again, these leaves were ground up and then applied to bee stings.

- **Wild Onion and Garlic**. The Dakotas and Winnebagos put the crushed bulbs of wild onions and garlic directly on the site of the sting.

Common Household Products for Sting Treatment

- Because **Witch Hazel** is a strong astringent, it causes contraction of the sting site. Although there is a relatively complicated concoction one can create with its leaves, twigs and bark, we will stick to the simpler version—the commercial one available just about anywhere. These products are not as strong, but they do have antiseptic, anesthetic and anti-inflammatory powers.

- **Cinnamon Oil** has been reported as a great natural pain killer because it acts as an anesthetic due to one of its ingredients, "eugenol." One would NOT apply it directly to the bite site, however. Cinnamon Oil can cause reactions of redness or burning, though it can be washed off if necessary. Cinnamon Powder has been found to stop bleeding and relax the muscles around the bite site. Again, a reaction may occur with this powder, so you should always wash and dry thoroughly if that happens.

- **Crushed garlic** is so versatile! Not only is it great for pesto and garlic bread, but it's a healthy and helpful substance. It's been called a "wonder drug" by many, and is advocated for treating many conditions, including hymenoptera stings.

Its claim to fame is its antibiotic properties, helping to ward off infection. In order for the garlic's qualities to be activated, the garlic must be crushed, chewed, chopped or otherwise in less than whole form.

Treat the bit topically with the crushed, mashed or minced garlic. You may ward off more than an infection with this remedy with the smell, but it could be well worth your while.

- **Saltbush**. The Navajos chewed the stems and placed the pulpy mash on areas of swelling caused by ant, bee and wasp bites. The Zunis applied the dried, powered roots and flowers mixed with saliva to ant bites.

- **Broom Snakeweed**. The Navajos used the resin from the stem to treat bites.

- **Tobacco**. Tobacco and tea leaves are both excellent neutralizers for the pain and swelling from insect stings. (See my own story on the next page for an illustration of this fact!) With teabags such a common item in most kitchens, we can be assured of having this particular remedy wherever we go.

- **Goldenseal** is a fairly well-known healing treatment these days and its uses are many. It seems that the Cherokees used the rootstock combined with bear fat to smear on their bodies as a general insect repellent.

A Wasp-y Story

A few years ago, I volunteered to be the first cleaner-upper in a large meeting hall that had been standing idle all winter. It was March and still quite chilly. The hall was completely empty but for a few chairs and tables. I zealously went to work, vacuuming and washing (maybe "zealously" is a tad of a stretch...). When I got to the corner of the room I reached down to pick up a crushed brown paper bag to throw away, but what I came away with was a hand full of wasp stings. These sleepy wasps had been happily dozing until I came along and woke them up before their winter was really over.

After screaming and carrying on for a while (there was no one to hear but the mice, I looked around for something to help the pain and swelling. The hall looked more barren than ever. I searched the kitchen area in the back to no avail. Nada, ziltch, niente, zip. I turned to return to my car to drive down the mountain to help (can you believe it, I was actually on the top of a mountain in this predicament!), when I spotted a lone teabag on the floor. I remembered reading somewhere that tea leaves were a great remedy for insect bites and stings. I pounced. I wet it with snow and shredded the tea leaves over my hand.

Within seconds my hand felt better and, though I was quite miserable for the next few days, I made it down the mountain without risking life and limb to get back safely to humanity.

Remember:

Always consult with your health care professional before using any new remedy.

The 10th Thing to Know

Bee-ing Careful & Consciencious

Pesticides & "Pest" Elimination

Do we really mean it when we call these flying forms of nature "pests?" Well, maybe they pester us just a little—especially if they sting us or invade our homes. But, fortunately, most of the time it's not necessary to destroy them let alone an entire colony of insects.

Let's not forget that bees and wasps are links in the chain of nature. From pollination to producing honey to eating garden pests for sustenance, these insects play an essential role. Yellow jackets are also considered beneficial around home gardens and commercially grown fruits and vegetables at certain times of the year because some of their favorite meals include caterpillars and harmful flies. It is true, however, that yellow jackets are known for their presence around beehives in fall and will enter and even rob honey if given the opportunity.

When and if you *do* decide that a nest or colony of bees or wasps needs destroying, please DO IT RIGHT. Calling in the experts is by far the best way to go.

The first thing to ask yourself is, "What time of year is this?" Because occupied nests will only remain occupied until the following autumn. If you can wait, if they're far away from your house or in the attic, for example, then wait until the nest is empty in the late autumn and seal up its entrance. If a nest is high up in a tree, I recommend ignoring it altogether!

ELIMINATION TIPS

- Never try to burn or flood a nest with water (or pour boiling water on it). Hymenoptera get very VERY angry and aggressive with that particular tactic. Not a good idea.

- If you do decide to destroy the nest yourself, use a product containing one of the following chemicals:

Baygon, pyrethirin, permethrin or resmethrin; or a natural trap method.

- Use a product (with the above chemicals) with a spray stream that shoots a lot at one time and FAR! You don't want to be anywhere near that nest when you start your siege.

- WAIT UNTIL AFTER DARK WHEN THE INSECTS HAVE RETURNED HOME from a hard day at work and have kicked their shoes off. It pays to wait.

- Completely saturate the nest to destroy those insects inside and those directly hit by the spray. Naturally, you try to make direct contact with as many as possible.

- Don't ever stand right under the nest. Just because you've taken down an insect, it can still sting for some time. Stay out of the way.

- Wasp nest in the garden? Some advocate eliminating it with diesel fuel or gasoline. This technique sounds pretty tough to us, so if you try it, *bee-ware* and *bee careful.*

We got this approach from a website (see *Resource* Pages). Fill an ordinary bottle with fuel. Always come at the nest entrance from the side—not the front or back. Never shine your flashlight on the nest because the guard wasps will surely be alerted and get a quick clue about the nature of your visit. The best time to attempt any kind of elimination is at dusk when you can still see, but the insects tend to have begun "relaxing" for the night. TIP: use a flashlight covered with red cellophane if you have to work at night. Yellow jackets are unable to see red.

Once you've opened the bottle, QUICKLY approach the nest entrance from the side. Again, make sure you keep your light away from the entrance—it only alerts the guard wasps. Uncork the bottle and swiftly ram the bottle (full of fuel) upside down into the entrance, completely eliminating the insects' only way out.

- Insect safe traps are now available also and we highly recommend this method if you have the time and patience. You simply insert a piece of bait into the trap to attrack the bees, wasps, etc., and then watch as they fly in and can't get out. You can even let them out somewhere far away...a perfectly *humane* thing to do.

- One educator recommends drenching the exit hole with an approved insecticide and then plugging the hole with treated soil or cotton balls. If not killed by this initial treatment, the wasps soon will be after chewing on the treated cotton ball or tunneling through the soil.

- Entrance holes in buildings are more easily handled with "dusts." Dust insecticide sticks to the insects' legs and goes with them back to their nests. Thus, grooming insects will eventually ingest the poison. Death of a colony may take up to a week and repeated chemical applications may be necessary.

ABSOLUTELY, POSITIVELY
DO NOT
IGNITE NESTS OR HIVES

Because nests have only one egress that serves as both the entrance and the exit, the entire nest's insect population will die from the gas's fumes alone over the next 24 to 36 hours. Ignition is unnecessary and dangerous.

Our Hornet Story

Recently, our 14-year-old son let us know in his inimitable fashion that we had a "hornet's nest in the our mailbox!" Well, all of a sudden my daily trips down to the mailbox, sticking my hand in to retrieve the mail, didn't look so appealing—I'm talking besides the usual daily arrival of bills.

My husband and I tromped down the driveway to check it out. Sure enough, a little hive stuck to the inside top of the box. Very little, but not little enough for me.

We convened and discussed the options. "Get the RAID," my son yelled. I was afraid he'd wake up every last wasp, hornet, and bee in the vicinity with that one.

My research at that point sure came in handy. "STOP," I instructed. "Hold evreything. We shouldn't try to destroy it until after dark when they're all back in their nest for the night."

"Really?" asked Joey, suspended mid-stride in disbelief. (14-year-olds are struck down more often by lightning than the belief that a parent might be knowledgable about anything.

So we waited a couple of hours, left the mail in the box, and then took the RAID down. We reassessed the situation and the angles, aimed the nozzle and then heavily sprayed the entire nest until it was saturated. The next day the nest was on the bottom of the box. We gave it a couple of more sprays and days and then removed it. *Total Success*.

AUTHORS' RECOMMENDATION:

Removing nests can be very dangerous. Again, our nest was a true "mini" of a nest. We would suggest that it is always best, whether you know you're allergic or just to be safe, whether you go the "trapping route" or not, to hire a professional exterminator for the job. You want it done right and you don't want to get hurt.

To our readers:

There is much, much more information on the topic of bees and other stinging insects we could impart, but, to be true to our "everything you need to know in about an hour" philosophy, we will stop here. We hope that the information you've learned will stand you in good stead to handle most things that come your way relative to stinging insects.

RELATED LINKS

1. Galaen.med.virginia.edu
   (Dr. Bower's Complimentary Medicine Home Page)
2. www.wvu.edu
   (W. Virginia University—article on wasp stings)
3. www.sparks.org
   (Sparks Healthcare System—on-line medical library)
4. www.ohioline.osu.edu
   (treating bee stings)
5. www.draperbee.com
   (apiary site)
6. www.beehivestore.com
7. www.intelihealth.com
   (article on avoidance and prevention)
8. www.mckinley.uiuc.edu
   (McKinley Health Center Web site—limited, but
   helpful information
9. www.primus.com/~spectrum/apitherapy.tuml
   (Spectrum Medical Arts: article by Dr. Glenn
   Rothfeld on BVT
10. www.allergysa.org
    (alalergic reactions to bees and wasps)
11. www.parenting.com (first aid for stings helpful to
    parents)
12. www.onehealth.com

13. www.insectstings.co.uk (individual's personal story, including his long illness andtreatment programs); David Glaser was kind enough to provide many of the photos for this book from his site.
14. www.hon.com (Healthcare Network Foundation: links to other resources)
15. www.acme.com/jef/
16. http://msa.ars.usda.gov/la/btn/hbb
17. www.angelfire.com/ok3/vespids/index.html (Benefits to humans from wasps and hornets)

RESOURCES

1. Medic Alert Foundation, 2323 Colorado Avenue, Turlock CA 95380. Tel: 1-800-922-3320.
2. The American Apitherapy Society, Inc., PO Box 54, Hartland Four Corners, VT 05049. Voice 1-800-823-3460. Fax 1-802-436-2827. International 1-802-436-2708.
3. American College of Allergy, Asthma & Immunology, 85 W. Algonquin Rd, Suite 550, Arlington Heights, IL 60005. Tel: 1-708-427-01200
4. ALK LAboratories, Inc., Wallingford, CT. For more information, call 1-800-325-7354

BOOKS of INTEREST

1. *Bees Don't Get Arthritis* by Fred Malone (Academy Books)
2. *Bee in Balance* by Amber Rose (Starpoint Ltd)

When Heidi Ratner-Connolly and Randy Connolly found themselves frustrated by the lack of down-to-earth, accessible information on topics that were of particular personal concern, they decided to write their own books to answer that need. It was then that 2LAKES PUBLISHING and the

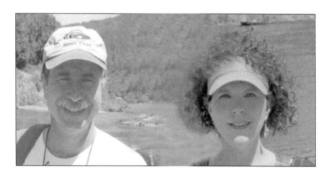

10 things to know™ series of books were born, generating books that are "long on information when you're short on time." The Connollys are dedicated to publishing books that help people live healthier, happier lives, and to living their own lives in the pursuit of a similar goal. They are currently living on the magnificent coast of Oregon.